Phobias and Fears

First Edition

Roy Basa

Edited by Marie Ezekiel
Graphic Artist and Cover Designer: Tess Ritumalta

Photos used are taken from google and may dontain its own copyright

ISBN:
Hardbound-978-621-470-330-2
MOBI/KINDLE-978-621-470-331-9
Softbound/Paperback-978-621-470-332-6

Published in the Philippines by:
Poetry Planet Book Publishing House
Rosario, Pozorrubio, Pangasinan, Philippines
Contact No.: 09554960044
Email: maritesritumalta@gmail.com

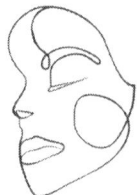

PREFACE

This book on Phobias and Fears is inspired by one of my classes as we do our classroom quiz bee on the different phobias and fears.

As their teacher, I prepared by researching the most common phobias and fears to be included in the said activity, but as I go along, I realized that I almost have all the phobias on the list, so I just realized that what if I will publish a book out of that simple activity?

It is the ultimate goal of this book to really make the definition of 480+ phobias as simple as possible for everybody to easily remember, learn and enjoy at the same time.

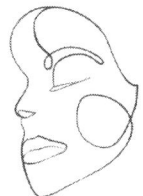

DEDICATION

This book is ultimately dedicated to my wife Rozel Jaena Basa, and to our children, Niel Michael, Jasper Miguel, and Amara Celestine.

Secondly, to my Tatay Raul Ornillo Basa, Nanay Lilia Pabiana Binas, and to all my siblings namely, Ricky, Rene, Cathy, Lilian, Raul Jr., and Jess Adel.

Lastly, to my classes, who participated in our classroom quiz bee on phobias and fears.

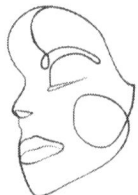

TABLE OF CONTENTS

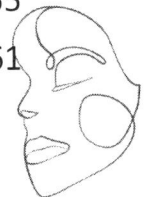

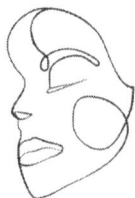

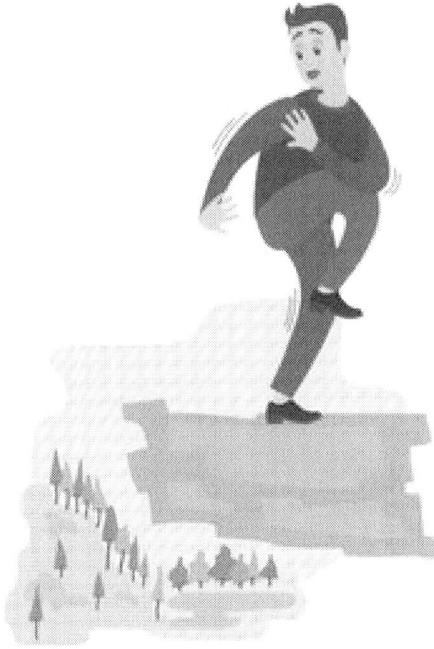

Acrophobia-fear of heights

A

Acrophobia	fear of heights
Agateophobia	fear of madness
Agoraphobia	fear of leaving the House
Algophobia	fear of pain
Allodoxaphobia	fear of what other people will say about him/her
Apiphobia	fear of stinging Insects
Aquaphobia	fear of drowning in Water
Arachnophobia	fear of spiders
Arsonphobia	fear of fire.
Asthenophobia	fear of fainting
Astrophobia	fear of celestial bodies, space, and stars.

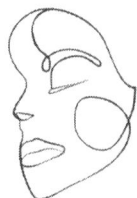

8

Astraphobia	fear of thunder
Astrapophobia	fear of thunder
Asymmetriphobia	fear of asymmetry
Ataxiophobia	fear of muscular incoordination or physical symptoms
Ataxophobia	fear of disorder or uncleanliness or untidiness
Atelophobia	fear of being unsystematic or ruin
Athazagoraphobia	fear of being ignored, forgotten, and unremembered
Atomosophobia	fear of explosion from atomic and nuclear bomb
Atychiphobia	fear of failure and being unsuccessful
Aulophobia	fear of flutes or orchestra

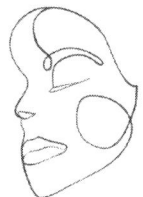

9

Aurophobia	fear of gold
Auroraphobia	fear of Aurora Borealis
Autodysomophobia	fear of one's foul body odor
Automatonophobia	fear of dummies, mannequins, wax statues, or diorama models
Automysophobia	fear of being dirty, germs, and being infected or contaminated
Autophobia	fear of being alone
Aviophobia	fear of riding any Vehicle

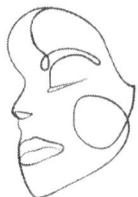

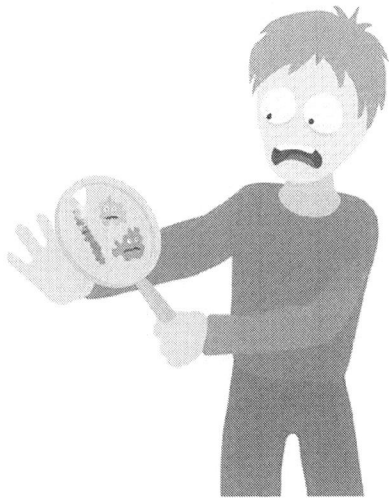

Bacillophobia-fear of microbes

B

Bacillophobia	fear of microbes
Bacteriophobia	fear of bacteria
Ballistophobia	fear of missiles and bullets
Bolshephobia	fear of Bolsheviks
Barophobia	fear of gravity
Basophobia	fear of walking or Falling
Bathmophobia	fear of stairs or sloppy structures
Bathophobia	fear of deep places or Structures
Batophobia	fear of being close to high buildings and structures
Batrachophobia	fear of amphibians
Belonephobia	fear of pins and Needles

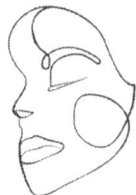

12

Bibliophobia	fear of books
Blennophobia	fear of slimy things
Bogyphobia	fear of bogeyman
Botanophobia	fear of plants
Brontophobia	fear of thunder, lightning and storms
Bufonophobia	fear of toads

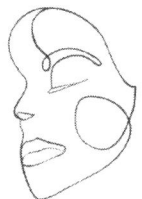

13

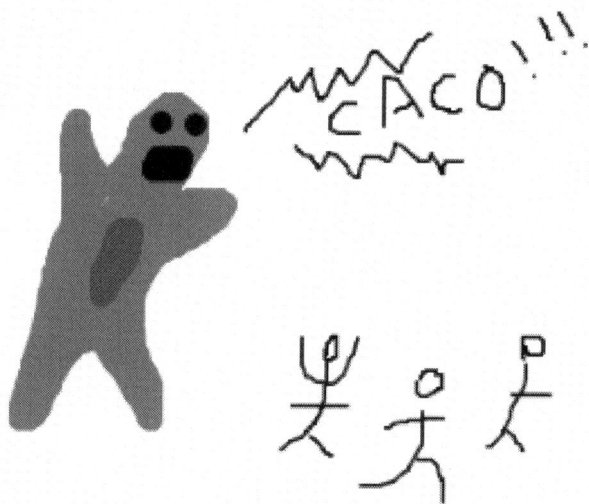

Cacophobia-fear of ugliness

C

Cacophobia	fear of ugliness
Cainophobia	fear of newness
Caligynephobia	fear of beautiful Women
Cancerophobia	fear of cancer
Carcinophobia	fear of cancer
Cardiophobia	fear of the heart
Carnophobia	fear of meat
Catagelophobia	fear of being laughed at or ridiculed
Catapedaphobia	fear of jumping
Cathisophobia	fear of mirrors
Cenophobia	fear of lightning
Ceraunophobia	fear of being unsuccessful/failures
Cheimaphobia	fear of cold

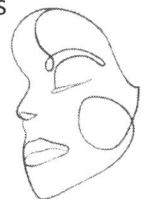

15

Chemophobia	fear of chemicals
Cherophobia	fear of gaiety
Chionophobia	fear of snow
Chiraptophobia	fear of being touch
Chirophobia	fear of hands
Chiroptophobia	fear of bats
Cholerophobia	fear of cholera
Chorophobia	fear of dancing
Chrometophobia	fear of money
Chromophobia	fear of time
Chronomentrophobia	fear of clocks
Cibophobia	fear of food
Claustrophobia	fear of confined Spaces
Cleptophobia	fear of stealing

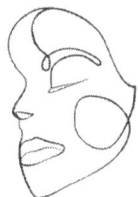

Climacophobia	fear of stairs, climbing and falling down
Clinophobia	fear of being Enclosed
Cnidophobia	fear of comets
Cometophobia	fear of colors
Coimetrophobia	fear of cemeteries
Coitophobia	fear of coitus
Contreitpphobia	fear of sexual abuse
Coprastasophobia	fear of constipation
Coprophobia	fear of feces
Consecotaleophobia	fear of chopsticks
Coulrophobia	fear of clowns
Counterphobia	fear of not finding the source of their phobia; seeking out the condition that is feared
Cremnophobia	fear of precipices

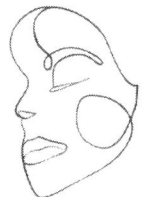

Cryophobia	fear of extreme cold
Crystallophobia	fear of crystals
Cyberphobia	fear of computers
Cyclophobia	fear of bicycles
Cymophobia	fear of waves or wavelike motions
Cynophobia	fear of dogs or rabies
Cypridophobia	fear of prostitutes

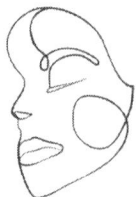

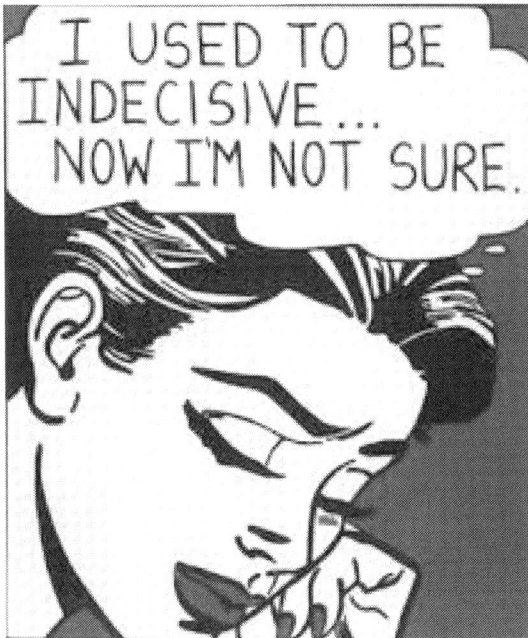

Decidophobia-fear of making decisions

D

Decidophobia	fear of making decisions
Defecaloesiophobia	fear of having a painful bowel movement
Deipnophobia	fear of dining conversation
Dementophobia	fear of insanity
Demonophobia	fear of demons
Demophobia	fear of crowds
Dentophobia	fear of dentists
Dermatophobia	fear of skin diseases
Dextrophobia	fear of objects on the right side of the body
Diabetophobia	fear of diabetes
Didaskaleinophobia	fear of going to school

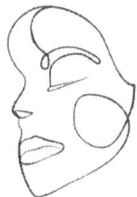

Dikephobia	fear of being right and just; justice
Dinophobia	fear of dizziness and whirlpools
Dipsophobia	fear of drinking
Dishailiophobia	fear of undressing
Disposophobia	fear of throwing out things
Domatophobia	fear of houses
Doraphobia	fear of fur
Doxophobia	fear of expressing oneself
Dromophobia	fear of crossing the street
Dutchphobia	fear of the Dutch
Dysmorphophobia	fear of deformity
Dystychiphobia	fear of accidents

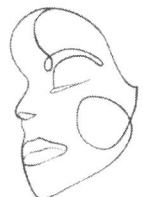

21

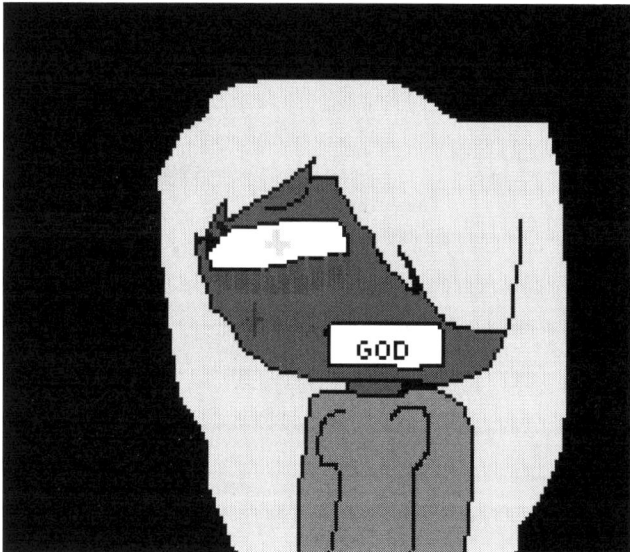

Ecclesiophobia-fear of going to church

E

Ecclesiophobia	fear of going to church
Ecophobia	fear of home
Eicophobia	fear of home surroundings
Eisoptrophobia	fear of one's image in the mirror
Electrophobia	fear of electricity
Eleutherophobia	fear of freedom
Elurophobia	fear of cats
Emetophobia	fear of vomiting
Enetophobia	fear of getting poked by a pin
Enochlophobia	fear of a chaotic environment
Enosiophobia	fear of criticism
Entomophobia	fear of bug bites

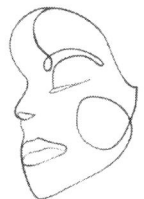

23

Eosophobia	fear of sunrise
Ephebiphobia	fear of teenagers
Epistaxiophobia	fear of nosebleed
Epistemophobia	fear of knowledge
Equinophobia	fear of horses
Eremophobia	fear of loneliness
Ereuthrophobia	fear of blushing
Ergasiophobia	fear of work
Erotophobia	fear of sexual love
Euphobia	fear of good news
Eurotophobia	fear of female genitalia
Erythrophobia	fear of color red

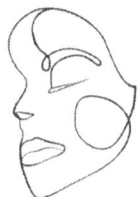

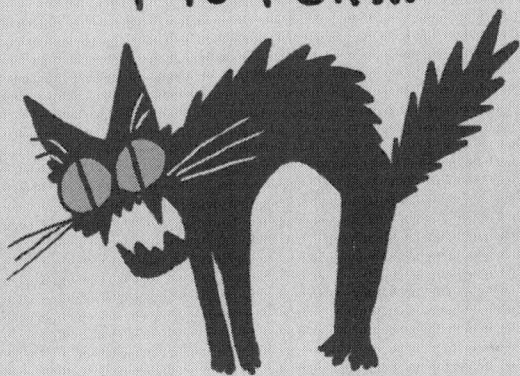

Felinophobia-fear of cats

f

Felinophobia   fear of cats

Febriphobia   fear of fever

Frigophobia   fear of cold things

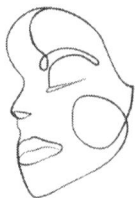

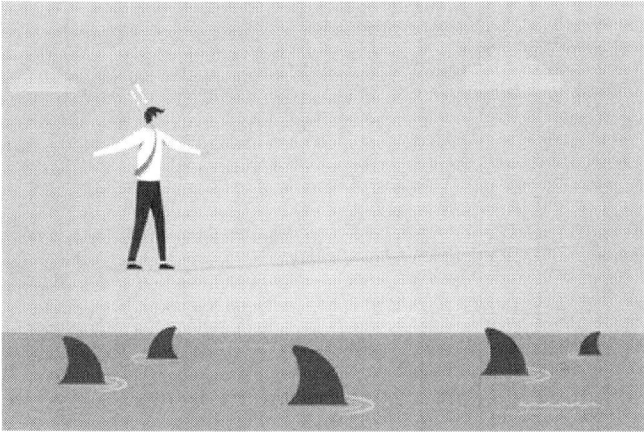

Galeophobia-fear of sharks

G

Galeophobia	fear of sharks
Gallophobia	fear of French culture
Gamophobia	fear of marriage
Geliophobia	fear of hearing laughter
Gelotophobia	fear of being laughed
Geniophobia	fear of chins
Genophobia	fear of sex
Genuphobia	fear of knees
Gephyrophobia	fear of crossing bridges
Germanophobia	fear of German culture
Gerascophobia	fear of growing
Gerontophobia	fear of growing old
Geumaphobia	fear of taste

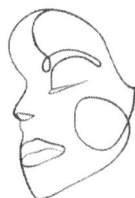

Glossophobia	fear of speaking in public
Globophobia	fear of balloons
Gnosiophobia	fear of knowledge
Graphophobia	fear of handwriting
Gymnophobia	fear of nudity
Gynephobia	fear of women

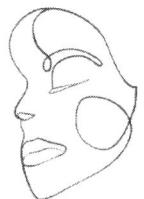

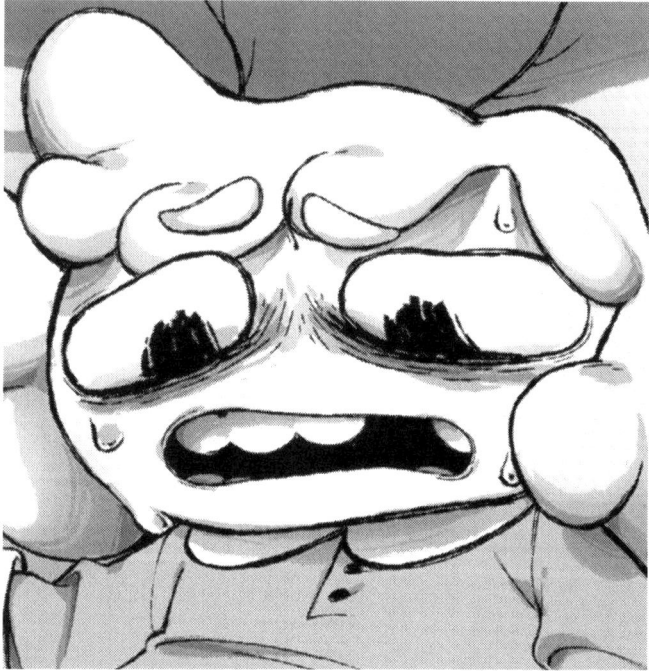

Hadephobia-fear of hell

H

Hadephobia	fear of hell
Hagiphobia	fear of saints or holy things
Hamartophobia	fear of committing sin
Haphephobia	fear of being touch
Harpaxophobia	fear of being robbed
Hedonophobia	fear of feeling happy
Heliophobia	fear of the sun
Hellennologiophobia	fear of the Greek
Helminthphobia	fear of the worm Infestation
Hemophobia	fear of blood
Heresyphobia	fear of radical deviation from official doctrine
Herpetophobia	fear of reptiles

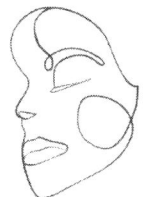

Heterophobia	fear of opposite sex
Hexakosioihexekontahexaphobia-fear of 666	
Hierophobia	fear of priest
Hippophobia	fear of horses
Hippopotomonstrosesquipedaliphobia-fear of long words	
Hobophobia	fear of beggars
Hodophobia	fear of traveling by road
Hormephobia	fear of death
Homichlophobia	fear of fog
Homilophoboia	fear of sermons
Hominophobia	fear of men
Homophobia	fear of homosexuality
Hoplophobia	fear of firearms
Hydrargyophobia	fear of mercurial Medicine
Hydrophobia	fear of water

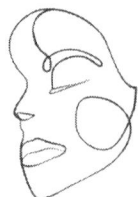

Hydrophobophobia	fear of rabies
Hyelophobia	fear of glass
Hygrophobia	fear of moisture
Hylephobia	fear of epilepsy
Hylophobia	fear of forests
Hypengyophobia	fear of responsibility
Hypnophobia	fear of sleep or being hypnotized
Hypsiphobia	fear of height

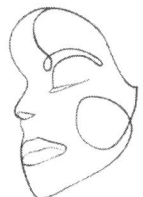

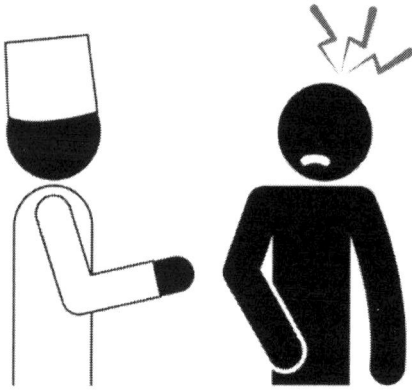

Iatrophobia-fear of physicians

I

Iatrophobia	fear of physicians
Ichthyophobia	fear of fish
Ideophobia	fear of idea
Illyngophobia	fear of vertigo
Iophobia	fear of poison
Insectophobia	fear of insects
Isolophobia	fear of isolation
Isopterophobia	fear of termites

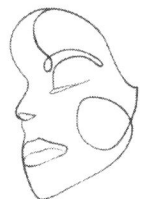

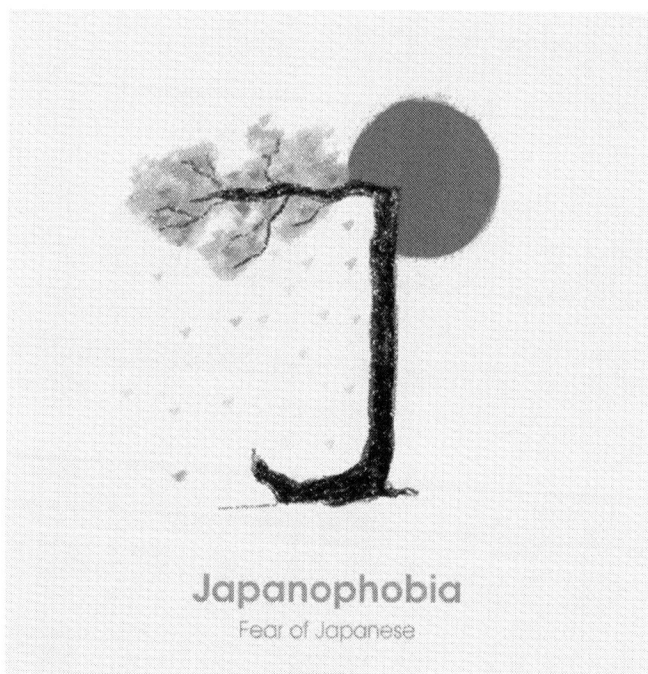

Japanophobia
Fear of Japanese

J

Japanophobia   fear of Japanese
                                     culture

Judeophobia   fear of the Jews

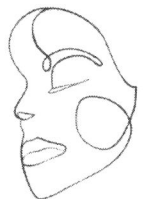

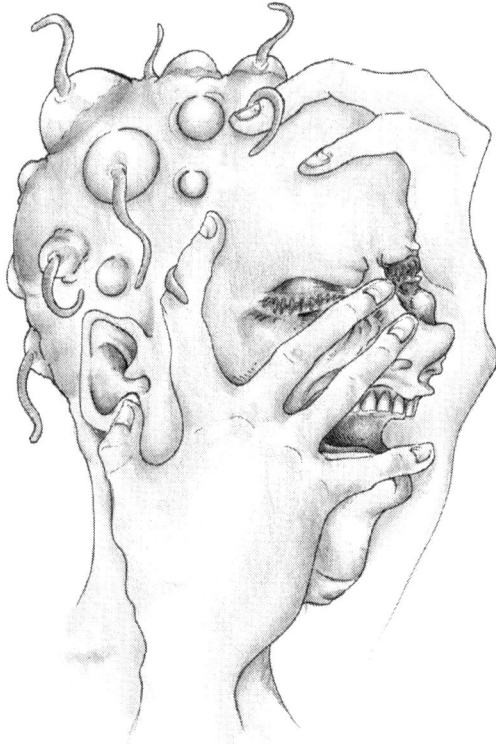

Kakorrhaphiophobia-fear of social media

K.

Kakorrhaphiophobia	fear of social media
Kainolophobia	fear of having a new or novel thing
Katagelophobia	fear of being embarrassed
Kathisophobia	fear of sitting down
Katsaridaphobia	fear of cockroaches
Kenophobia	fear of empty space
Keraunophobia	fear of storms, thunder, and lightning
Kinetophobia	fear of movement
Kleptophobia	fear of stealing
Koinoniphobia	fear of rooms
Kolpophobia	fear of female genitals
Kopophobia	fear of fatigue

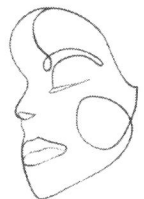

Koniophobia	fear of dust
Kosmikophobia	fear of the cosmic phenomenon
Koumpounophobia	fear buttons
Kymophobia	fear of waves
Kyphophobia	fear of stooping

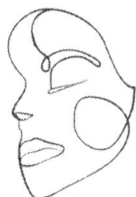

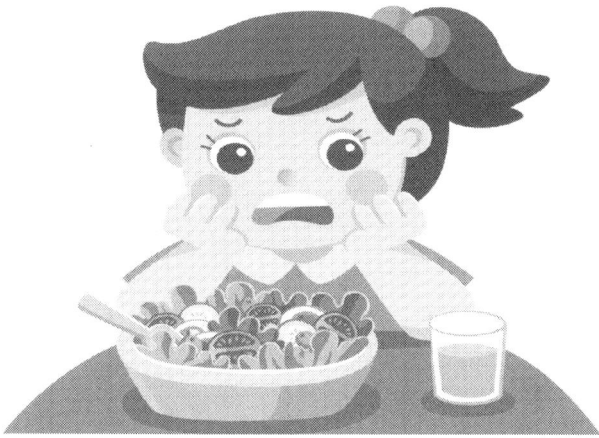

Lachanophobia-fear of vegetables

L.

Lachanophobia	fear of vegetables
Laliophobia	fear of humanity
Lepidopterophobia	fear of butterflies
Leprophobia	fear of leprosy
Leukophobia	fear of color white
Levophobia	fear of things from the left side of the body
Ligrophobia	fear of loud noise
Lilapsophobia	fear of tornadoes and hurricane
Limnophobia	fear of lakes
Linonophobia	fear of strangulation
Liticaphobia	fear of lawsuits
Lockiophobia	fear of childbirth
Logizomechanophobia	fear of computers

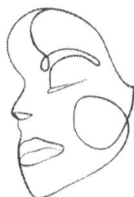

Logophobia	fear of words
Luiphobia	fear of flu and communicable disease
Lutraphobia	fear of otters
Lygophobia	fear of darkness
Lyssophobia	fear of rabies

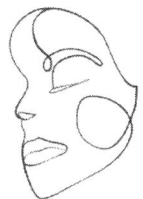

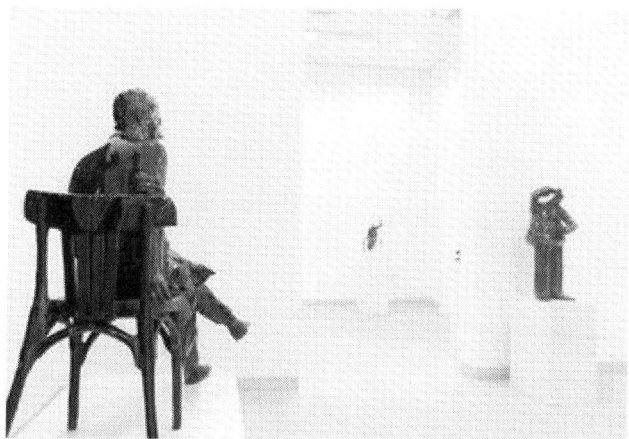

Macrophobia-fear of long waits

M

Macrophobia	fear of long waits
Mageirocophobia	fear of cooking
Maieusiophobia	fear of childbirth
Malaxophobia	fear of love – play
Maniaphobia	fear of insanity
Mastigophobia	fear of punishment
Mechanophobia	fear of machines
Medomalacuphobia	fear of losing an erection
Medorthophobia	fear of an erect penis
Megalophobia	fear of large things
Melissophobia	fear of bees
Melanophobia	fear of the color black
Melophobia	fear of music
Meningitophobia	fear of brain disease

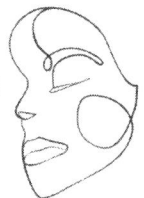

45

Menophobia	fear of menstruation
Merinthophobia	fear of challenges
Metallophobia	fear of metal
Metathesiophobia	fear of change
Meteorophobia	fear of cosmic proportions
Methyphobia	fear of alcohol
Metrophobia	fear of poetry
Microbiophobia	fear of microbes
Microphobia	fear of small things
Mysophobia	fear of memories
Molysmophobia	fear of dirt contamination
Monophobia	fear of isolation
Motorphobia	fear of automobiles
Mottephobia	fear of moths

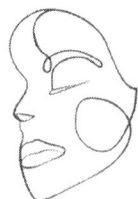

Musophobia	fear of mice
Mycophobia	fear of mushrooms
Mycrophobia	fear of very small things
Myctophobia	fear of darkness
Myrmecophobia	fear of ants
Mythophobia	fear of myths
Myxophobia	fear of slimy things

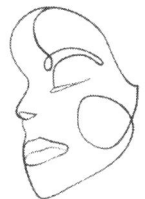

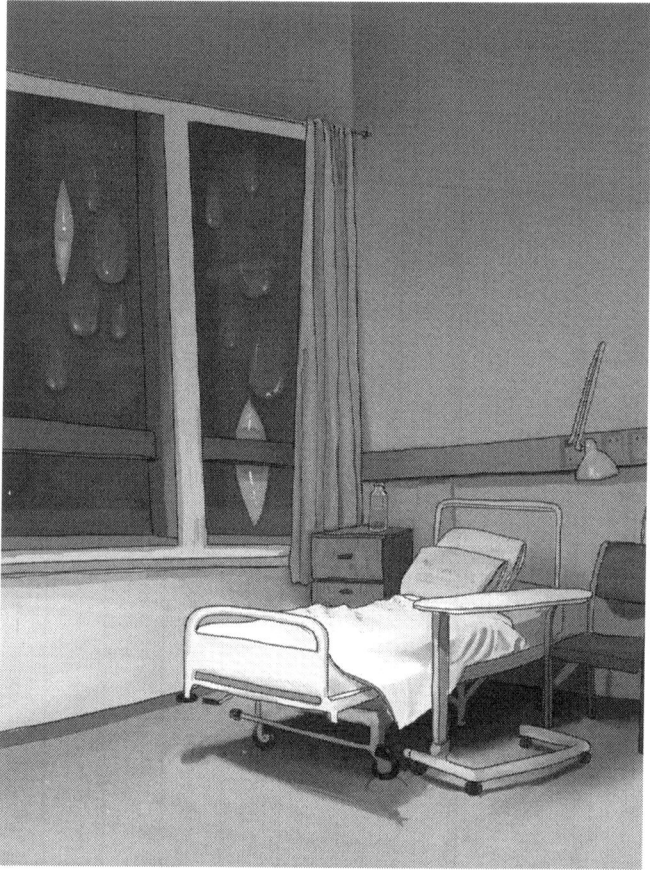

Necrophobia-fear of dead things/funerals

N

Necrophobia	fear of dead things/funerals
Nebulaphobia	fear of fog
Nelophobia	fear of glass
Neopharmaphobia	fear of new drugs
Neophobia	fear of anything new
Nephophobia	fear of clouds
Noctiphobia	fear of nighttime
Nomatophobia	fear of names
Nosocomephobia	fear of hospitals
Nosophobia	fear of a definite disease
Nostophobia	fear of returning home
Novercaphobia	fear of step-mother

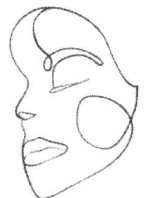

49

Nucleomituphobia	fear of the nuclear weapon
Nudophobia	fear of nudity
Numerophobia	fear of numbers
Nyctohylophobia	fear of dark wooded areas
Nyctophobia	fear of darkness and unknown

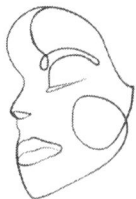

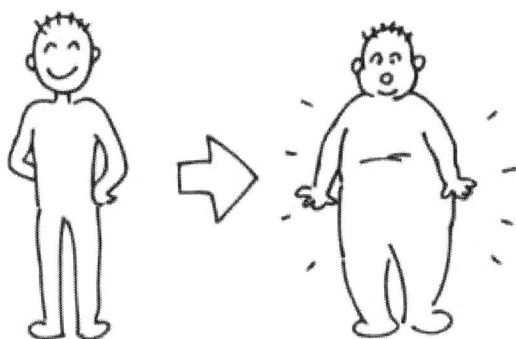

Obesophobia-fear of gaining weight

O

Obesophobia	fear of gaining weight
Ochlophobia	fear of crowds
Ochophobia	fear vehicles
Octophobia	fear of figure eight
Odontophobia	fear of dental surgery or falling teeth
Odynophobia	fear of pain
Oenophobia	fear of wines
Oikophobia	fear of home surroundings
Olfactophobia	fear of smells
Ombrophobia	fear of rain
Ommetaphobia	fear of eyes looking at you
Omphalophobia	fear of belly buttons
Oneirophobia	fear of dreams

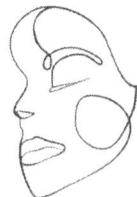

Oneirogmophobia	fear of wet dreams
Onomatophobia	fear of hearing
Ophidiophobia	fear of snakes
Ophthalmophobia	fear of being stared
Opiophobia	fear of doctor's prescription on pain medication
Optophobia	fear of opening one's eyes
Ornithophobia	fear of birds
Orthophobia	fear of property
Osmophobia	fear of smells
Ostraconophobia	fear of shellfish
Ovophobia	fear of eggs
Ouranophobia	fear of heaven

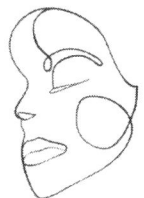

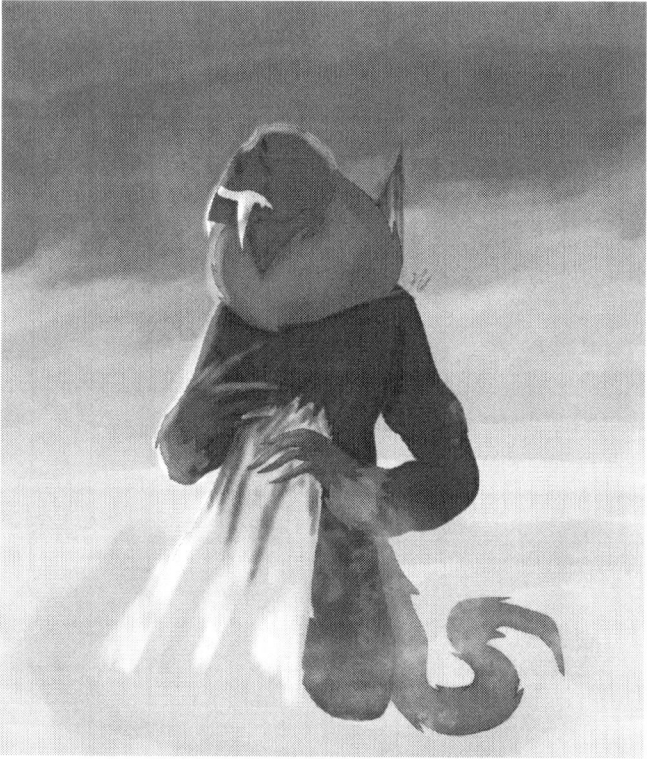

Pagophobia-fear of extreme cold

P

Pagophobia	fear of extreme cold
Panthophobia	fear of suffering too much pain
Panophobia	fear of everything
Papaphobia	fear of the Pope
Papyrophobia	fear of paper products
Paralipophobia	fear of being corrupted
Paralipophobia	fear of neglecting duty
Paraphobia	fear of being corrupted by sexual perversion
Parasitophobia	fear of parasites
Paraskavedekatriaphobia	fear of Friday the 13th
Parthenophobia	fear of virgins

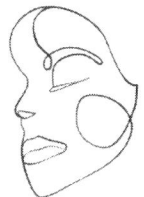

Pathophobia	fear of disease
Patroiophobia	fear of heredity
Parturiphobia	fear of pregnancy or childbirth pain
Peccatophobia	fear of sinning or imagery crimes
Pediculophobia	fear of extreme cold
Pediophobia	fear of dolls
Pedophobia	fear of children
Peladophobia	fear of bald people
Pellagrophobia	fear of pellagra
Peniaphobia	fear of poverty
Parthenophobia	fear of mother-in-laws
Phagophobia	fear of choking
Phalacrophobia	fear of becoming bald
Pharmacophobia	fear of taking medicine

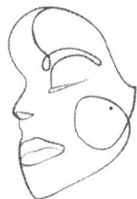

Phasmophobia	fear of ghosts
Phengophobia	fear of the light of day
Philemaphobia	fear of kissing
Philophobia	fear of falling in love or being in love
Philosophobia	fear of philosophy
Phobophobia	fear of phobias
Photoaugliaphobia	fear of glaring lights
Photophobia	fear of light
Phonophobia	fear of noises
Phronemophobia	fear of thinking
Phthiriophobia	fear of extreme cold, ice, or frost.
Placophobia	fear of tombstones
Plutophobia	fear of wealth
Pluviophobia	fear of rain

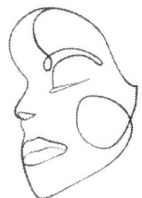

Pneumatiphobia	fear of spirits
Pnigophobia	fear of choking
Pocrescophobia	fear of gaining weight
Podophobia	fear of feet
Pogonophobia	fear of men with beards
Poliosophobia	fear of acquiring poliomyelitis
Politophobia	fear of politicians
Polyphobia	fear of being afraid
Poinephobia	fear of punishment
Ponophobia	fear of overworking
Porphyrophobia	fear of purple color
Portaphobia	fear of outhouses or port-a-potty
Potamophobia	fear of rivers

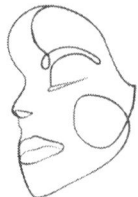

Potophobia	fear of losing control through alcohol intake
Proctophobia	fear of rectums
Prosophobia	fear of progress
Psellismorphobia	fear of stuttering
Psychphobia	fear of questioning oneself
Psychrophobia	fear of being freezing to death
Pteromerhanophobia	fear of flying
Pupaphobia	fear of puppets
Pyrexiophobia	fear of fever
Pyrophobia	fear of fire

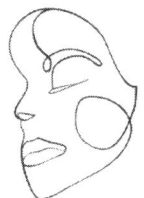

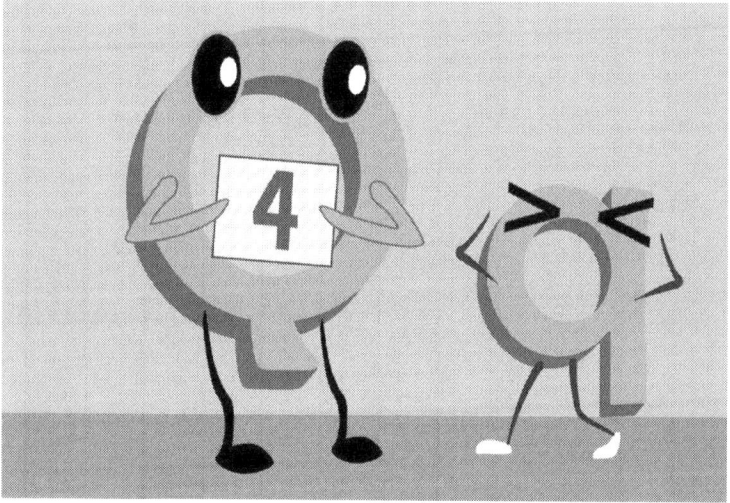

Quadraphobia-fear of number 4

Q

Quadraphobia	fear of number 4
Quadriplegiphobia	fear of being a quadriplegic
Quintaphobia	fear of number 5

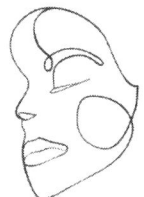

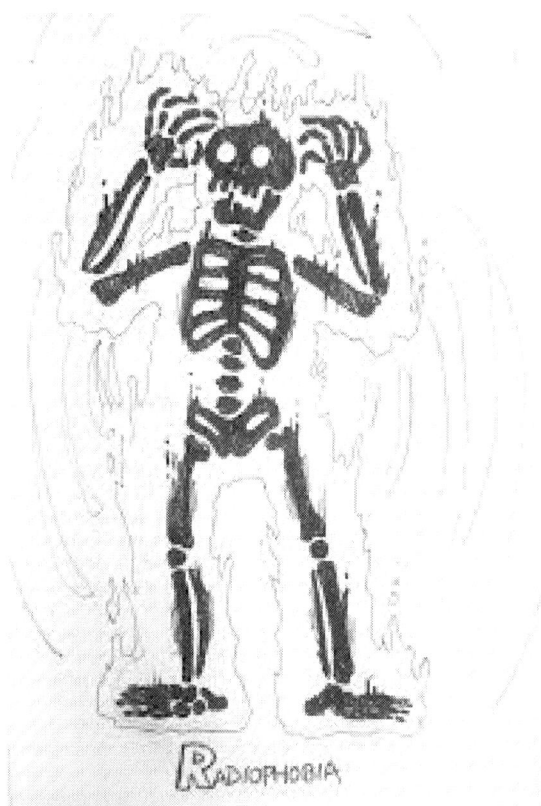

Radiophobia-fear of radiation and x- rays

R

Radiophobia	fear of radiation and x- rays
Ranidaphobia	fear of frogs
Rectophobia	fear of rectum
Rhabdophobia	fear of being severely punished
Rhypophobia	fear of defecation
Rhytiphobia	fear of getting wrinkles
Rophobia	fear of trees
Rupophobia	fear of dirt
Russophobia	fear of Russians

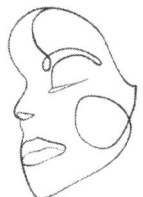

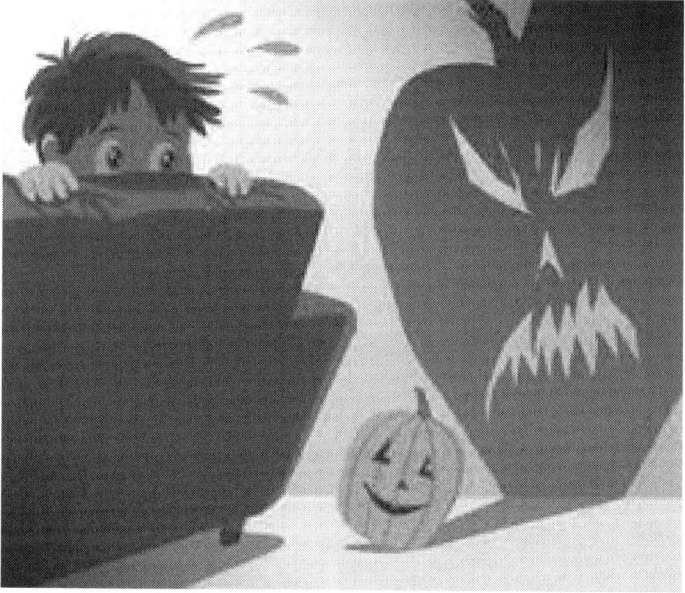

Samhainophobia-fear of Halloween

S

Samhainophobia	fear of Halloween
Sarmassophobia	fear of love-play
Satanophobia	fear of Satan
Scabiophobia	fear of scabies
Scatophobia	fear of fecal matter
Sciophobia	fear of shadows
Scoleciphobia	fear of worms
Scolionophobia	fear of school
Scopophobia	fear of being seen or starred
Scotomaphobia	fear of blindness
Scotophobia	fear of darkness
Scriptophobia	fear of public writing
Selachophobia	fear of sharks
Selenophobia	fear of the moon

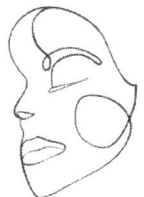

Seplophobia	fear of decaying matter
Sesquipedalophobia	fear of long words
Sexophobia	fear of the opposite gender
Siderodromophobia	fear of trains
Siderophobia	fear of stars
Sidonglobophobia	fear of cotton balls
Sinistrophobia	fear of being left-handed
Sinophobia	fear of Chinese
Sitophobia	fear of food
Snakephobia	fear of snake
Soceraphobia	fear of parents-in-law
Social phobia	fear of being evaluated negatively in social areas.
Sociophobia	fear of society

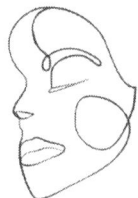

Somniphobia	fear of sleep
Sophophobia	fear of learning
Soteriophobia	fear of dependence on others
Spacephobia	fear of the outer space
Spectrophobia	fear of ghost
Spermatophobia	fear of germs
Spheksophobia	fear of wasps
Stasibasiphobia	fear of standing or walking
Staurophobia	fear of crucifix
Stenophobia	fear of narrow things
Styglophobia	fear of ending up in hell
Suriphobia	fear of mice
Symbolophobia	fear of symbolism
Symmetrophobia	fear of symmetry

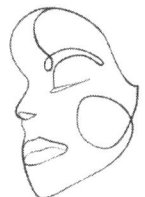

Syngenesophobia   fear of relatives

Syphilophobia   fear of syphilis

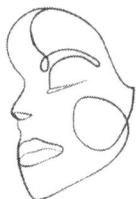

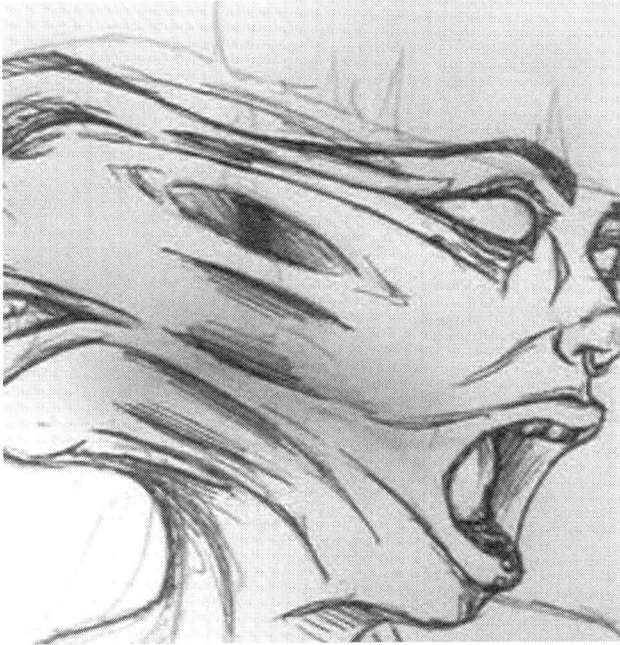

Tachophobia-fear of speed

T

Tachophobia	fear of speed
Taeniophobia	fear of tapeworms
Taphephobia	fear of being buried alive
Tapinophobia	fear of being contagious
Taurophobia	fear of bulls
Technophobia	fear of technology
Teleophobia	fear of liturgy and rigid laws
Telephonophobia	fear of the telephone
Teratophobia	fear of bearing a deformed child
Testophobia	fear of taking tests
Tetanophobia	fear of tetanus
Teutophobia	fear of the Germans

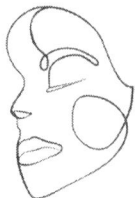

Textophobia	fear of fabrics
Thaasophobia	fear of being seated
Thalassophobia	fear of a vast world
Thanatophobia	fear of death
Theatrophobia	fear of theaters
Theologicophobia	fear of God
Theophobia	fear of theology
Thermophobia	fear of heat
Thyphallophobia	fear of having an erect penis
Tocophobia	fear of childbirth
Tomophobia	fear of surgical operations
Tonitrophobia	fear of thunder
Topophobia	fear of certain places or situations
Toxiphobia	fear of poison

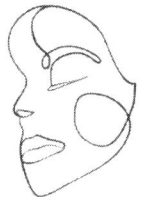

Traumatophobia	fear of injury
Tremophobia	fear of degenerative disease
Trichinophobia	fear of parasites
Trichopathophobia	fear of hair
Triskaidekaphobia	fear of number 13
Tropophobia	fear of moving
Trypanophobia	fear of injections
Trypophobia	fear of small holes
Tuberculophobia	fear of tuberculosis
Tyrannophobia	fear of tyrants
Uranophobia	fear of heaven
Urophobia	fear of urine or urination

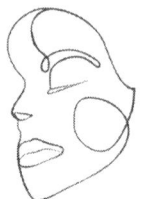

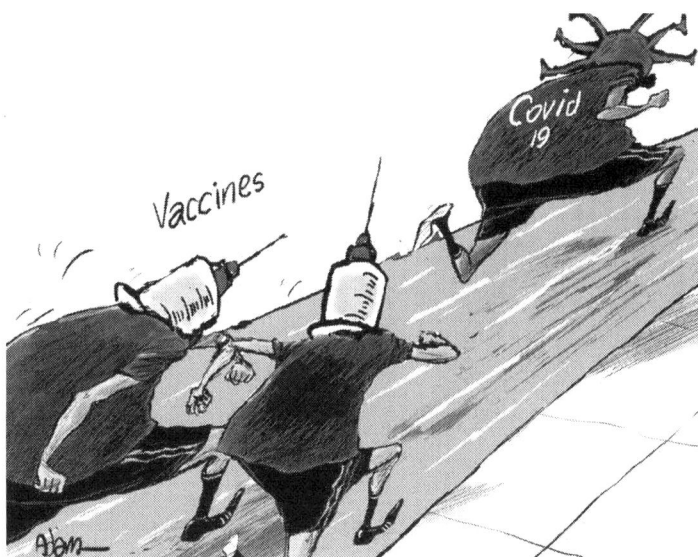

Vaccinophobia-fear of vaccination

V

Vaccinophobia	fear of vaccination
Venustraphobia	fear of beautiful women
Verbophobia	fear of words
Vehophobia	fear of driving
Verminophobia	fear of germs
Vestiphobia	fear of clothing
Virginitiphobia	fear of step-father

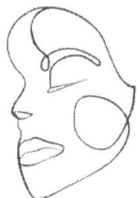

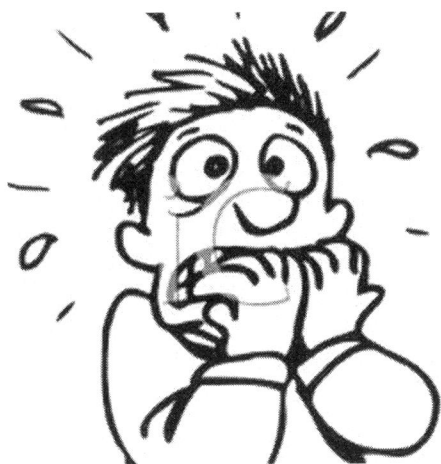

Walloonphobia-fear of Walloons

W

Walloonphobia   fear of Walloons

Wiccaphobia   fear of witches and
witchcraft

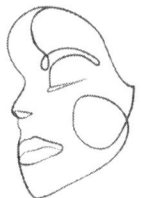

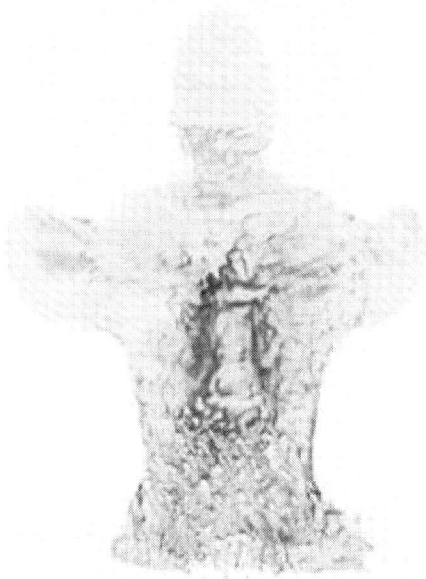

Xanthophobia-fear of color yellow

X

Xanthophobia	fear of color yellow
Xenoglossophobia	fear of foreign language
Xenophobia	fear of strangers
Xerophobia	fear of dryness
Xylophobia	fear of things made up of wood
Xyrophobia	fear of razors

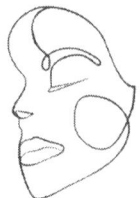

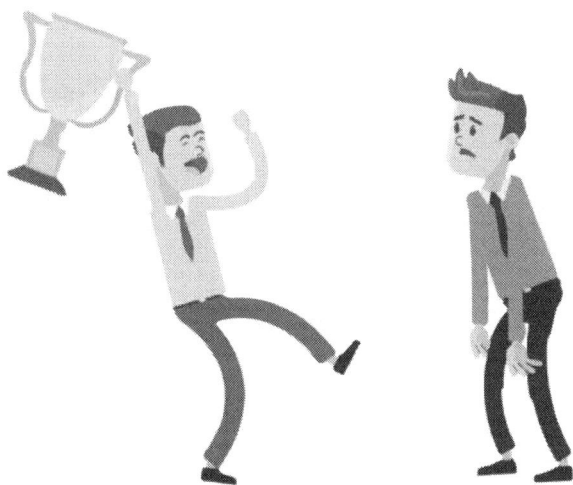

Zelophobia-fear of jealousy

Z

Zelophobia   fear of jealousy

Zeusphobia   fear of gods

Zemmiphobia   fear of the mole

Zoophobia   fear of animals

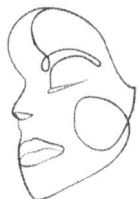

ABOUT THE AUTHOR

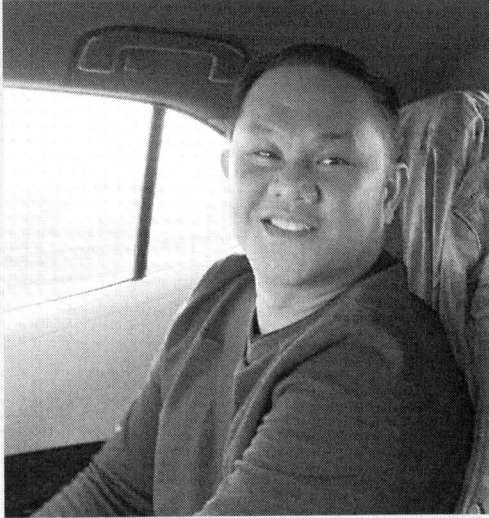

ROY B. BASA,
LPT, Ph.D., DHum,
DMinEd, DSc, FOPd, FRIEdr

    Roy Basa was born and raised in Murcia, Negros Occidental, Philippines by Raul and Lilia Basa together with his other 6 siblings. He graduated his elementary education from Lopez Jaena Elementary School. He then went to La Consolacion College, Murcia for his secondary education where he graduated as Class Valedictorian of 1998. He got his Bachelor's in Education major in General Science, Masters in School Administration and Supervision, and Doctor of Philosophy major in Educational Management at

University of Negros Occidental – Recoletos where he graduated with Outstanding in Dissertation and High Academic Excellence Awards. He then took another masterate, the Master in Natural Science at University of St. La Salle, Bacolod under a scholarship grant, Project – Free Paglaum.

He was a high school, college, and graduate school science teacher for 18 years in the Philippines and 3 years as high school science and career technical education (CTE) teacher in Arizona and New Mexico, USA, respectively.

He was awarded as one of the Most Outstanding Teachers of the Philippines in 2016 by the Metrobank Foundation. Recently, he was also awarded by 6th Asia – Pacific Luminare Awards as "Asia's Most Remarkable and Exceptional Science and CTE Educator of the Year 2022.

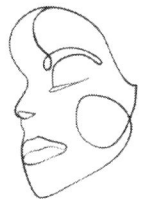

Made in the USA
Las Vegas, NV
13 October 2022